Keto Diet Cookbook for Beginners

Quick & Easy Ketogenic Recipes to Lower Cholesterol and Lose Weight for living healthy

Stephanie Robbins

information contained within this document, including, but not limited to, errors, omissions, or inaccuracies.

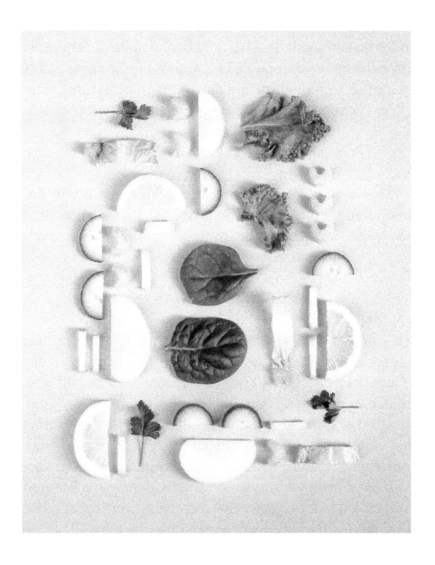

Table of Contents

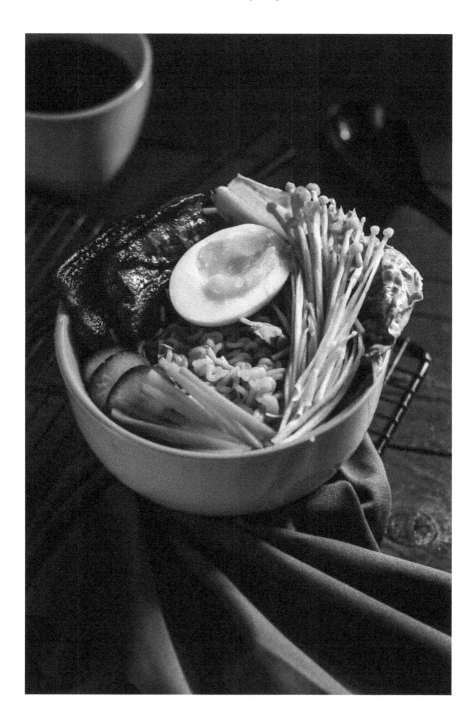

Introduction

A t first, the keto diet is very simple. It is a diet where the person is required to stop eating foods that contain lots of carbs (sugar) and start eating foods that have high-fat content.

Keto diet is mostly associated with high protein intake. While people are aware that it is possible to achieve weight loss through the keto diet only, the majority of them are not aware that it is possible to build muscles with the help of keto. Getting your muscles in shape is fun with keto. It does not matter if you are male or female you can achieve what you want with keto.

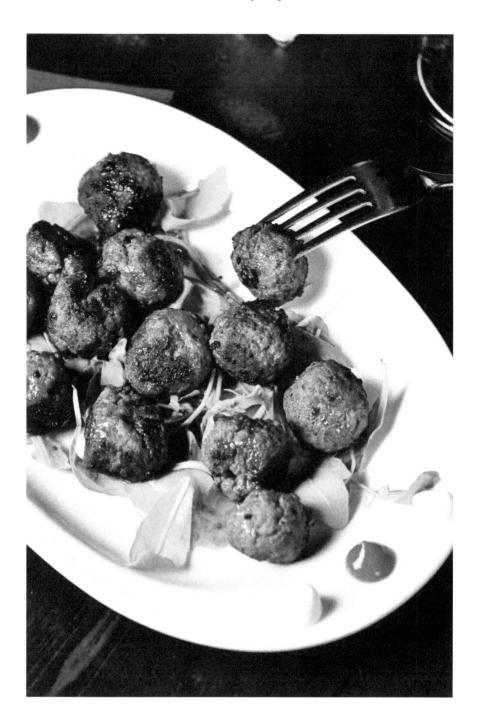

The **Keto** Diet

Although going on a keto diet offers a lot of benefits, it is important to know about what you are getting into. As a woman over her fifties, it is essential to know all the necessary to overcome challenges and achieve your long-term goal.

There will be a radical change in the way you are currently eating. The typical or standard diet is particularly high in carbohydrates, and diving into a keto diet could prove very difficult. People who adopt the ketogenic diet certainly get a series of benefits. However, before starting, you need to prepare yourself mentally, knowing, and following all the essential guidelines.

Know what to eat and avoid while on the keto diet

The meal plan for a keto diet aims to reduce carbs drastically. According to Kristen Mancinelli, a dietician based in New York and the author of The Ketogenic Diet: A Scientifically Proven Approach to Fast, Healthy Weight Loss, You can begin with an amount of 20 to 30 grams of carbohydrates every day.

You also have to know carb-rich foods, protein, and fat. This enables you to choose the foods that will keep you on a ketogenic diet wisely. You may think that only foods such as pasta, cookies, bread, ice-cream, and candy are rich in carbs. Although, for example, beans have some proteins, it is a food that is rich in carbohydrates, too. Also, many vegetables and fruits have high carbohydrate content. Foods that contain little or no carb include pure fats, butter, oils, and meat.

Know your relationship with fatty food

As a woman above 50, this is an important aspect that can't be overlooked. According to Mancinelli, the common belief of many people is that the intake of fat can kill them. Another unclear point about this is that there is currently no conclusive result in support or against this belief. According to some researches, eating polyunsaturated fats instead of saturated is essential to reduce the risk of heart disease. On the other hand, many other research studies point to the fact that total fat and various types of fats are not related to cardiovascular diseases. This controversy makes choosing what to eat a little confusing. Despite all these confusions, it is essential to note that as a woman over 50, the food you eat contains far more than one nutrient. Therefore, the important is the total quality of the diet, although more research is still needed to determine the risk and health benefits of keto.

In situations where you should eat potatoes or rice in your meal, you can instead choose a non-starchy vegetable. When cooking, you can start using more oil, such as avocado or olive oil. You will have to do away with old dieting habits. You can't just go to make a grilled plain-looking skinless chicken breast, as this doesn't make sense when on keto. That is because it doesn't contain enough fat.

Foods to Eat

The Good Fats

Add Extra-Virgin Olive Oil (EVOO): Olive oil dates back centuries to a time where oil was used for anointing kings and priests.

Add Macadamia Oil: One of the benefits of this oil is its high smoke point of 390° Fahrenheit. It carries a mild flavor, which is a super alternative for olive oil in mayonnaise.

Other Monounsaturated & Saturated Fats: Include these items (listed in grams):

- Organic red palm oil, Avocado, Sesame, Olive, & Flaxseed Oil - Unsalted butter, Chicken fat, Duck fat, & Beef tallow (1 tbsp. = 0 g net carbs)

- Ghee (1 tsp. = 0 g net carbs)

- Olives (3 jumbo - 5 large/10 small = 1 g net carb)

- Unsweetened flaked coconut (2 tbsp.=3 g net carbs)

Dairy & Your Diet

Before beginning the keto way of life, you need to understand dairy and dairy products, which are an essential part of the ketogenic methods. If you're lactose intolerant, maybe the plan isn't for you. The amounts should be monitored to no more than four ounces daily. Choose dairy products that have been cultured and are keto-friendly. The number one choice is unsweetened almond milk. You can also choose from hemp milk and flax milk.

Calcium

- **Broccoli rabe—cooked:** 3.5 ounce portion = 120 mg per 100 grams

- **Greens (spinach, kale, etc.) cooked:** 3.5 ounce portion = 135 mg per 100 grams

- **Sesame seeds:** 1 ounce portion = 273 mg per 28 grams

- **Almond milk (calcium-fortified):** 8 ounce portion = 300-450 mg per 225 grams

- **Almonds:** 1 ounce portion = 74 mg per 28 grams

Omega 3 Fatty Acids Options

Alpha-linoleic acid (ALA) is the most common omega-3 fatty acid in your diet. The acid content is found in these using one tablespoon portions:

- **Chia Seeds:** 2.5 grams per 14-gram portion

- **Ground Flaxseed:** 1.6 grams per 7-gram portion

- **Hemp Seeds:** 2 grams per 20-gram portion

Iron Options

Be sure you have adequate iron in your diet. Include these food groups:

- **Cooked spinach:** 3.5 ounce portion = 3.6 mg per 100 grams

- **Cooked white mushrooms:** 3.5 ounce portion = 2.7 mg per 100 grams

- **Olives:** 3.5 oz. portion = 3.3 mg per 100 grams

- **Sesame seeds:** 1 ounce portion = 4.1 mg per 28 grams

- **Pumpkin seeds:** 1 ounce portion = 4.2 mg per 28 grams

- **Chia seeds:** 1 ounce portion = 2.2 mg per 28 grams

- **Coconut milk:** 3.5 oz. portion = 3.3 mg per 100 grams

- **Canned hearts of palm:** 3.5 oz. portion = 3.1 mg per 100 grams

- **Dark chocolate:** 1 ounce portion = 3.3 mg per 28 grams

Save Additional Carbohydrates

- **Pasta:** Replace pasta using zucchini. Use a spiralizer and make long ribbons to cover your plate. It is excellent for many dishes served this way. You can also prepare spaghetti squash for regular spaghetti.

- **French Fries:** Change over to zucchini fries or turnip fries.

- **Tortillas:** Get ready to push this one to the side, which weighs in at approximately 98 grams for one serving. Instead, enjoy a lettuce leaf at about 1 gram per serving.

- **Mashed Potatoes:** There's no need to prepare bowls of regular mashed potatoes; instead, enjoy some mashed cauliflower.

-

Foods to Avoid

The Limited "Bad" Fats

You need to be aware of unhealthy, processed trans fats, and polyunsaturated fats. These fats are acquired through processing and are found in foods, including fast foods, crackers, margarine, and cookies. Avoid canola, soybean, safflower, and cottonseed vegetable oils. If the oil was processed in a factory and prepackaged, you need to be aware of its fat content.

Processed Foods

Don't purchase any items if you see carrageenan on the label. Like so many other people, you shouldn't feel too guilty if you crave all of those processed foods. It happens!

Generally, look for labels with the least amount of ingredients. Usually, the ones that provide the most nutrition are listed in those shorter lists.

Here are just a few of the items you may not realize are loaded with carbs:

Watch out for the Sugar Products also:

- **Raw Sugar:** 12 grams of carbs

- **High-Fructose Corn Syrup:** 14 grams of carbs

- **Honey:** 17 grams of carbs

- **Maple Syrup:** 14 grams of carbs

- **Cane Sugar:** 12 grams of carbs

Some of the foods are surprising because they were deemed for years as a healthy and nutritious snack. I bet you see a few of the culprits that will beckon you onto the wrong path:

- Cereal Bars

- Rice Cakes

- Protein Bars

- Potato Chips

- Flavored Nuts

- Popcorn

- Pretzels

- Crackers

Benefits of Keto Diet

Now, we get to the reason we are all here! What is it that the ketogenic diet can do for you? Luckily for you, there are a number of benefits this new lifestyle can bring to you. Whether you are looking to lose weight, balance your hormones, or just be healthier overall, the ketogenic diet may be your best option!

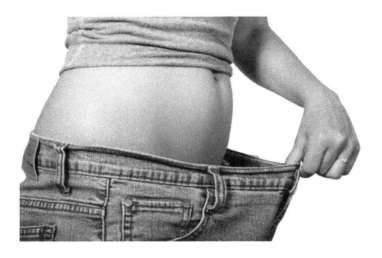

Weight Loss

Weight loss is one of the major reasons people begin the ketogenic diet in the first place. The idea of a high-fat, low-carb diet has been used for a very long time now. One of the major reasons the ketogenic diet works is due to the fact that this way of eating helps suppress appetite. As you lower your insulin levels by eating less carbs, you will be lowering the levels of fat in your body.

As you follow the ketogenic diet, you will be tapping into your own fat reserves as energy. Up until this point, your body has been using the easiest way to create energy from what it is given. From this point on, you will be retraining your body to use fat as energy instead! It is a win-win situation for you as you begin to feel more energetic and burn fat at the same time. As you do this and combine with ketone supplements, you will be losing weight in no time.

Lower Blood Sugar for Type 2 Diabetes

As mentioned earlier, the ketogenic diet can help individuals lower their insulin levels. This is due to the fact that your body will be running off ketones instead of relying on glucose. As your body learns how to utilize fat and ketones for energy, this means that you will no longer need to worry about excess blood sugar levels or the need to get exogenous insulin.

PCOS: Polycystic Ovary Syndrome

There are many women who suffer from PCOS. This syndrome is often linked to insulin resistance and in turn, causes a range of different hormonal issues for women. When following the ketogenic diet, this could help address the insulin resistance within the body and help those who have

PCOS. In one particular study, they found that the ketogenic diet did help improve body weight, testosterone markets, fasting insulin, and the LH/FSH ratio for the women who had PCOS.

IBS: Irritable Bowel Syndrome

If you have IBS, you may think that a high-fat, low-carb diet could mean doom for you. If you suffer with symptoms such as bloating, stomach discomfort, or chronic diarrhea, the ketogenic diet may be able to actually help you in the long run! The long-term effects may be worth it if you are on the fence about the diet.

At first, upping fat can cause a bit of increased diarrhea, but as you lower your sugar consumption, this may help provide relief to symptoms caused by IBS. In fact, individuals have claimed that the ketogenic diet can improve stool habits, abdominal pain, and improves the overall quality of life thanks to a proper diet!

Increased Brain Function

While weight loss is a popular reason individuals begin the ketogenic diet, another major reason is improved brain function. Think about it; how often do you have a hard time focusing on simple tasks? Perhaps you go through your day, feeling exhausted, and leaning on high-carb foods to get you through. What if I told you that that high-sugar, high-carbohydrate foods were doing you more harm than good? Sure, they give you a burst of energy, but then they make you tired all over again AND make you fat. Through the ketogenic diet, you can improve your ability to learn, improve your memory recollection, and improve overall brain function.

According to Dr. Myhill, he found that through the ketogenic diet, the heart and the brain are able to run up to 25% more efficient when the body is running on ketones as opposed to blood sugar. In a study done on older adults following the ketogenic diet, they were able to improve their overall memory function, including their short term memory.

Increased Mitochondrial Function

Let's take a moment and go back to high school science. As you recall, the mitochondria are the energy factories in your cells. If the cells did not have the mitochondria, we would all be dead. This is why the health of your mitochondrial function is vital for your health, performance, immune function, and more. We are only as healthy as our mitochondria. Luckily on the ketogenic diet, you can increase the function of your mitochondria!

According to Dr. Gabriela Segura, she explains that the mitochondria functions better on the ketogenic diet due to the fact that the diet has the ability to increase energy levels in a more efficient way that is both stable and long-burning. Through diet, you gain the ability to increase energetic output while reducing the production of the free radicals that can be damaging to your system.

You see, the mitochondria were designed to specifically use fat for energy in the first place. As you use fat as the energy source, this helps decrease the toxic load and increase energy production. The key here is fat metabolism through ketone bodies by the liver. This process can only occur within your mitochondrion, which stimulates powerful anti-inflammatory antioxidants in your body. As you increase the overall health of your mitochondria, you will increase the health of your whole body!

Stabilize Energy Levels

Let me paint you a picture. You are sitting at your desk, and the clock strikes noon. At this point, your morning coffee begins to wear off, and you begin craving a little pick-me-up. That is your body craving energy and running out of glucose to run off of. As you begin to follow a ketogenic diet, you can say goodbye to your cravings for sugar and caffeine. While following a proper diet, you can keep your energy levels stable throughout the day and avoid the mid-afternoon slumps you may be experiencing at this point.

When your body is running on ketones, this is a readily available source of energy. As your body adapts to using this new source of energy, you will easily be able to get through your day without having energy level swings or food for that matter! Through consuming fewer calories, you can still lose weight and feel energetic at the same time!

Athletic Performance

The ketogenic diet is a very popular option for athletes due to enhanced endurance performance. While there have been many studies done on ketosis and sports performance, one, in particular, is known as the FASTER study. The results of this study showed that for those who followed a ketogenic diet, they had more mitochondria compared to the control group. This meant that these individuals had lower lactate load, lower oxidative stress, and were fueled off fat for a higher-intensity workout.

Alzheimer's

As more research is being completed on the ketogenic diet, scientists are starting to believe that the ketogenic diet could have a major effect on those who have Alzheimer's. In fact, some scientists refer to this disease as Type 3 diabetes due to the fact that as this happens, the brain loses its ability to utilize glucose, leading to high levels of inflammation. While this poses as an issue, under the proper diet, the brain could still be able to function on ketones. It is still being studied closely, but it could be a step in the proper direction.

Cancer

Another growing belief in the science community is that ketosis could be a key prevention of cancer. This may be due to the fact that cancer cells survive on glucose as a fuel source. On the ketogenic diet, individuals deprive the cancer cells of the glucose in the first place and can starve out the cancer in the process. While it is still being studied, it is becoming more popular for individuals who are being treated for several different types of cancer.

While these are some of the major benefits of the ketogenic diet, the list can go on for a very long while and is becoming longer as researchers complete more studies of the diet to have a better understanding. The ketogenic diet can also benefit:

- Heartburn

- Fatty Liver Disease

- Migraines

- Mood Stabilization

- Parkinson's Disease

Breakfast Recipes

1. Low Carb Caesar Salad

Preparation Time: 20 minutes

Cooking Time: 0 minutes

Servings: 4

Ingredients:

- 1 head romaine lettuce
- 6 slices cooked and diced bacon
- ½ cup shredded parmesan cheese
- 5 tablespoons grated parmesan cheese
- 3 teaspoons Worcestershire sauce
- 2 teaspoons fresh lemon juice
- 2 minced anchovy fillets, or anchovy sauce
- 2/3 cup Keto mayonnaise
- ¼ cup sour cream
- 1 minced garlic clove
- 1 teaspoon mustard powder
- Black pepper

Directions:

1. Slice the lettuce, and mix with the cheese and bacon like a normal salad.

2. For the dressing, put all the ingredients in a single bowl and mix well.

3. Set down your salad and top with as much dressing as you want. Enjoy!

Nutrition:

- Calories: 112 kcal

- Total Fat: 32g

- Total Carbs: 5.0g

- Protein: 14.3g

2. Keto Cauliflower and Eggs
Preparation Time: 20 minutes

Cooking Time: 5 minutes

Servings: 4

Ingredients:

- 5 hard-boiled eggs
- 2 stalks celery
- 1 ½ cups Greek yogurt
- ¼ teaspoon pepper
- 1 head cauliflower
- 1 tablespoon white vinegar
- 1 tablespoon yellow mustard
- 1 teaspoon salt
- 1 cup water
- ¾ white onion, diced

Directions:

1. Chop the cauliflower into bite-size pieces, and place it in a pot with a cup of water.

2. Drain the cauliflower and set aside

3. Dice up the boiled eggs, mix them into the cauliflower.

4. Dice the celery and onion, and then add in the cauliflower and egg mixture.

5. Add the Greek yogurt, pepper, white vinegar, yellow mustard salt, and the diced white onion to the mixture, and mix well with a wooden spoon.

6. Dish with salt and serve.

Nutrition:

- Calories: 224 kcal

- Total Fat: 22g

- Total Carbs: 8.2g

- Protein: 23.5 g

3. Zucchini Pizza Bites

Preparation Time: 30 minutes

Cooking Time: 10 minutes

Servings: 4

Ingredients:

- 4 large zucchinis
- 1 cup tomato sauce
- 2 teaspoon oregano
- 4 cups mozzarella cheese
- ½ cup parmesan cheese
- Low carb pizza toppings of your choice

Directions:

1. Slice your zucchinis into small pieces, in a quarter of an inch or less.

2. Preheat the oven to 450°F.

3. Line a baking pan or tray with foil, set it aside.

4. Place zucchini pieces in the pan. Top them with tomato sauce, cheese, oregano, and other low carb toppings you like. Bake for five minutes, and then broil for five minutes more. Serve warm.

Nutrition:

- Calories: 231 kcal Protein: 26.7g
- Carbs: 4.8g Fat:: 74g

4. Egg on Avocado

Preparation Time: 20 minutes Cooking Time: 5 minutes Servings: 3

Ingredients:

- 1 ½ teaspoon garlic powder
- ¾ teaspoons sea salt
- 1/3 cup Parmesan cheese
- ¼ teaspoon black pepper
- 4 avocados
- 6 small eggs

Directions:

1. Preheat muffin tins to 350°F.

2. Slice the avocado into half, and take the seed out. Mix the pepper, salt, and garlic well.

3. Generously season your avocado with the above seasoning mix. Place the seasoned avocado in the muffin tin; side with the empty hollow facing up.

4. Whisk the egg and gently pour in each avocado. If you doubt that the avocado has enough space, lightly scrape the inside. Finally, sprinkle cheese on top of the avocado. Repeat the process for all, and then bake for 15 minutes and Serve hot.

Nutrition: Calories: 364 kcal Total Carbs: 2.5g Total Fat: 55.5g Protein: 13.5g

5. Keto Meatballs

Preparation Time: 30 minutes

Cooking Time: 20 minutes

Servings: 3

Ingredients:

- 11 eggs
- 7 ounces mozzarella cheese
- 4 ounces chopped and cooked bacon
- 3 chopped scallions
- 1 ounce ground beef
- Salt
- Pepper
- A teaspoon olive oil

Directions:

1. Preheat the oven to 350°F and grease the muffin tray with oil.
2. Put the scallions evenly in the tin at the bottom.
3. In a bowl, mix the eggs and add a teaspoon of oil.
4. Add in the cheese, salt and pepper to taste. Mix well.
5. In another bowl, mix the bacon and the chicken together.
6. Add this meat mixture into cheese and stir well until combined.

7. Pour the mix into the muffin tray and bake for 17-20 minutes.

8. Serve hot.

Nutrition:

- Calories: 632 kcal

- Fat: 43g

- Carbohydrates: 15g

- Protein: 49g

6. Keto Scrambled Eggs

Preparation Time: 10 minutes

Cooking Time: 5 minutes

Servings: 41

Ingredients:

- 3 eggs
- 1 ounce ghee
- Salt and pepper

Directions:

1. Whisk the eggs, then add salt and pepper to taste. Mix well.

2. Heat the oil in a skillet and pour in the egg mixture and scramble until you cook the eggs.

3. Serve hot.

Nutrition:

- Calories: 148 kcal
- Fat: 15g
- Carbohydrates: 1.3g
- Protein: 12g

7. Keto Flaxseed Bread

Preparation Time: 1 hour

Cooking Time: 35 minutes

Servings: 6

Ingredients:

- 7 egg whites
- 2 egg yolks
- 6 tablespoons coconut oil or olive oil
- 3 cups flaxseed
- 3 sachets Stevia
- 3 teaspoons baking powder
- 1 teaspoon salt
- ½ cups water

Directions:

1. Preheat the oven to 350°F.
2. Pour in the egg whites, egg yolks, flaxseed, Stevia, oil, salt, water, and baking powder in a mixing bowl, and mix well with a wooden spoon.
3. Put into a blender and blend for 2-3 minutes. You can use a hand mixer too.
4. Grease a baking pan and line it with parchment paper.
5. Pour the batter into the pan, and bake for 30 minutes.

6. Take out from the oven and let it cool on a cake rack before slicing it.

Nutrition:

- Calories: 199 kcal

- Total Fat: 39g

- Total Carbs: 8g

- Protein: 15g

8. Keto Omelet

Preparation Time: 10 minutes

Cooking Time: 5 minutes

Servings: 1

Ingredients

- 3 large eggs
- Salt and pepper
- ½ ounce butter
- 4 sliced mushrooms
- ½ ounce olive oil
- 1 ounce shredded parmesan cheese
- 1 small chopped onion

Directions:

1. Whisk the eggs and season with salt and pepper, then mix well.
2. Heat the oil or butter in a frying pan.
3. Add in the mushrooms and onions and sauté until onions become soft.
4. Pour in the egg mixture.
5. When the egg mixture is firm, then sprinkle cheese on top.
6. When the bottom is cooked, flip with a spatula, cook from another side.

7. Take out the omelet on a serving plate and enjoy.

Nutrition:

- Calories: 550 kcal
- Fat: 37g
- Carbohydrates: 06.7g
- Protein: 24g

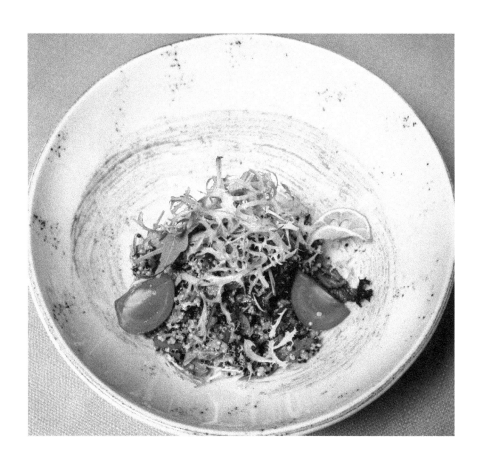

Lunch Recipes
9. Fish and Leek Sauté

Preparation Time: 15 minutes **Cooking Time:** 10 minutes **Servings:** 2

Ingredients:

- 1 leek, chopped

- 2 trout fillets, diced (approximately 8 oz.)

- 1 tablespoon tamari soy sauce

- 1 teaspoon ginger, grated

- 1 tablespoon avocado oil

- Salt to taste

Directions:

1. Over moderate heat in a large skillet; heat the avocado oil until hot. Once done; add and sauté the chopped leek for a few minutes, until turn soften.

2. Immediately add the diced trout with grated ginger, tamari sauce, and salt to taste.

3. Continue to sauté the trout until it's not translucent anymore and cooked through.

4. Serve immediately and enjoy.

Nutrition: Calories: 175 kcal Total Fat: 7.6g Saturated Fat: 1.5g Total Carbohydrates: 5.2g Dietary Fiber: 0.8g Sugars: 1.7g Protein: 21g

10. Keto Rib Eye Steak

Preparation Time: 5 minutes

Cooking Time: 20 minutes

Servings: 2

Ingredients:

- ½ pound grass-fed rib-eye steak, preferably 1" thick
- 1 teaspoon Adobo Seasoning
- 1 tablespoon extra-virgin olive oil
- Pepper and sea salt, to taste

Directions:

1. Add steak in a large-sized mixing bowl and drizzle both sides with a small amount of olive oil. Dust the seasonings on both sides; rubbing the seasonings into the meat.

2. Let sit for a couple of minutes and heat up your grill in advance. Once hot; place the steaks over the grill, and cook until both sides are cooked through (15 to 20 minutes) flipping occasionally.

Nutrition:

- Calories:257 kcalTotal Fat: 19g
- Saturated Fat: 5gTotal Carbohydrates: 0.3g
- Dietary Fiber: 0.2gSugars: 0g
- Protein: 24g

11. Eggless Salad
Preparation Time: 5 minutes

Cooking Time: 5 minutes

Servings: 4

Ingredients:

- 1 stalk celery, chopped
- Vegan mayonnaise, as required
- 1 pound extra firm tofu
- 2 tablespoons onions, minced
- Pepper and salt, to taste

Directions:

1. Mash the tofu into a chunky texture, just like an egg salad.
2. Add the mayonnaise until you get your desired consistency.
3. Add in the leftover ingredients; stir well.
4. Serve on keto pitas or keto bread, with vegetables and enjoy.

Nutrition:

- Calories: 117 kcalTotal Fat: 7.8g
- Saturated Fat: 1.3gTotal Carbohydrates: 2.8g
- Dietary Fiber: 1.5gSugars: 1.4g
- Protein: 16g

12. Mouth-Watering Guacamole
Preparation Time: 5 minutes

Cooking Time: 0 minutes

Servings: 6

Ingredients:

- 3 avocados, pitted
- ¼ cup cilantro, freshly chopped, plus more for garnish
- Juice of 2 limes
- ½ teaspoon kosher salt
- 1 small jalapeño, minced
- ½ small white onion, finely chopped

Directions:

1. Combine the avocados with cilantro, lime juice, jalapeño, onion, and salt in a large-sized mixing bowl; mix well.

2. Give the ingredients a good stir and then, slowly turn the bowl; running a fork through the avocados. Once you get your desired level of consistency, immediately season it with more salt, if required. Just before serving; feel free to garnish your recipe with more fresh cilantro.

Nutrition: Calories: 165 kcalTotal Fat: 15gSaturated Fat:: 2.1g Total Carbohydrates: 9.5g Dietary Fiber: 6.9g Sugars: 1.1g Protein: 2.1g

13. Smoked Salmon Salad

Preparation Time: 5 minutes

Cooking Time: 0 minutes

Servings: 1

Ingredients:

- 2 ounces smoked salmon
- 1 lemon slice
- 4 olives
- 1 teaspoon pink peppercorns, crushed lightly
- 1 handful arugula salad leaves, fresh

Directions:

1. Place the olives and salad leaves into a large plate or shallow bowl.

2. Arrange the smoked salmon over the salad.

3. Sprinkle the top of smoked salmon with lightly crushed pink peppercorns.

4. Garnish your salad with a lemon slice; serve immediately and enjoy.

Nutrition:

- Calories: 149Total Fat: 5.2g
- Saturated Fat: 1.4gTotal Carbohydrates: 4g
- Dietary Fiber: 1.7gSugars: 3.4g
- Protein: 11g

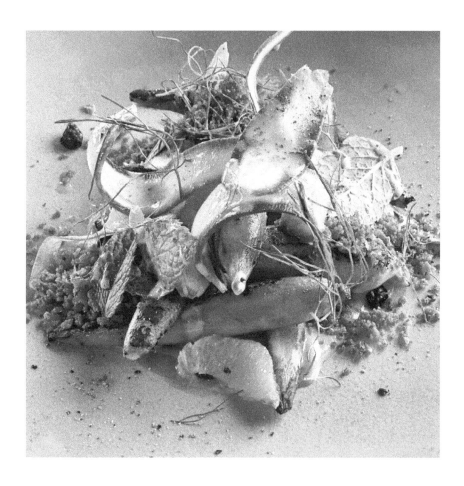

Dinner Recipes

14. Parmesan-Crusted   Halibut   with Asparagus

Preparation Time: 10 minutes

Cooking Time: 15 minutes

Servings: 4

Ingredients:

- 2 tablespoons olive oil

- ¼ cup butter, softened

- Salt and pepper

- ¼ cup grated Parmesan

- 1 pound asparagus, trimmed

- 2 tablespoons almond flour

- 4 (6 ounces) boneless halibut fillets

- 1 teaspoon garlic powder

Directions:

1. Preheat the oven to 400°F and line a foil-based baking sheet.

2. Throw the asparagus in olive oil and scatter over the baking sheet.

3. In a blender, add the butter, Parmesan cheese, almond flour, garlic powder, salt and pepper, and mix until smooth.

4. Place the fillets with the asparagus on the baking sheet, and spoon the Parmesan over the eggs.

5. Bake for 10 to 12 minutes, and then broil until browned (2 to 3 minutes).

Nutrition:

- Calories: 415 kcal

- Fat: 26g

- Protein: 42g

- Carbohydrates: 6g

- Fiber: 3g

- Net Carbs: 3g

15. Hearty Beef and Bacon Casserole
Preparation Time: 25 minutes

Cooking Time: 30 minutes

Servings: 8

Ingredients:

- 8 slices uncooked bacon
- 1 medium head cauliflower, chopped
- ¼ cup canned coconut milk
- Salt and pepper
- 2 pounds ground beef (80% lean)
- 8 ounces mushrooms, sliced
- 1 large yellow onion, chopped
- 2 cloves garlic, minced

Directions:

1. Preheat the oven to 37°F.
2. Cook the bacon in a skillet until it crisp, then drain and chop on paper towels.
3. Bring to boil a pot of salted water, and then add the cauliflower.
4. Boil until tender for 6 to 8 minutes then drain and add the coconut milk to a food processor.
5. Mix until smooth, then sprinkle with salt and pepper.

6. Cook the beef until browned in a pan, and then cut the fat away.

7. Remove the mushrooms, onion, and garlic, and then move to a baking platter.

8. Place on top of the cauliflower mixture and bake for 30 minutes.

9. Broil for 5 minutes on high heat, then sprinkle with bacon to serve.

Nutrition:

- Calories: 410 kcal

- Fat: 25.5g

- Protein: 37g

- Fiber: 3g

16. Sesame Wings with Cauliflower

Preparation Time: 5 minutes **Cooking Time:** 30 minutes **Servings:** 4

Ingredients:

- 2 ½ tablespoons soy sauce

- 2 tablespoons sesame oil

- 1 ½ teaspoons balsamic vinegar

- 1 teaspoon minced garlic

- 1 teaspoon grated ginger

- Salt

- 1 pound chicken wing, the wings itself

- 2 cups cauliflower florets

Directions:

1. In a freezer bag, mix the soy sauce, sesame oil, balsamic vinegar, garlic, ginger, and salt, then add the chicken wings. Coat flip, and then chill for 2 to 3 hours.

2. Preheat the oven to 400°F and line a foil-based baking sheet. Spread the wings along with the cauliflower onto the baking sheet. Bake for 35 minutes, and then sprinkle on to serve with sesame seeds.

Nutrition: Calories: 400 kcalFat: 28.5grotein: 31.5gCarbohydrates: 4gFiber: 1.5gCarbs: 2.5g

17. Fried Coconut Shrimp with Asparagus

Preparation Time: 15 minutes

Cooking Time: 10 minutes

Servings: 6

Ingredients:

- 1 ½ cups shredded unsweetened coconut
- 2 large eggs
- Salt and pepper
- 1 ½ pounds large shrimp, peeled and deveined
- ½ cup canned coconut milk
- 1 pound asparagus, cut into 2-inch pieces

Directions:

1. Pour the coconut onto a shallow platter.
2. Beat the eggs in a bowl with a little salt and pepper.
3. Dip the shrimp into the egg first, and then dredge with coconut.
4. Heat up coconut oil over medium-high heat in a large skillet.
5. Add the shrimp and fry over each side for 1 to 2 minutes until browned.
6. Remove the paper towels from the shrimp and heat the skillet again.

7. Remove the asparagus and sauté to tender-crisp with salt and pepper, and then serve with the shrimp.

Nutrition:

- Calories: 535 kcal
- Fat 38.5 g
- Protein: 29.5g
- Carbs: 18g
- Fiber: 10g
- Net Carbs: 8g

18. Chicken Tikka with Cauliflower Rice
Preparation Time: 10 minutes

Cooking Time: 6 hours

Servings: 6

Ingredients:

- 2 pounds boneless chicken thighs, chopped
- 1 cup canned coconut milk
- 1 cup heavy cream
- 3 tablespoons tomato paste
- 2 tablespoons Garam masala
- 1 tablespoon fresh grated ginger
- 1 tablespoon minced garlic
- 1 tablespoon smoked paprika
- 2 teaspoons onion powder
- 1 teaspoon guar gum
- 1 tablespoon butter
- 1 ½ cup rice cauliflower

Directions:

1. Place the chicken in a slow cooker and then stir in the remaining ingredients, except for the butter and cauliflower.

2. Cover and cook for 6 hours on low heat until the chicken is cooked and the sauce is thickened.

3. Melt the butter over medium to high heat into a saucepan.

4. Remove the riced cauliflower, and cook until tender (6 to 8 minutes).

5. Serve cauliflower rice with chicken Tikka.

Nutrition:

- Calories: 485 kcal

- Fat: 32g

- Protein: 43g

- Fiber: 1.5g

- Net carbs: 5g

19. Grilled Salmon and Zucchini with Mango Sauce

Preparation Time: 5 minutes

Cooking Time: 10 minutes

Servings: 4

Ingredients:

- 4 (6 ounces) boneless salmon fillets

- 1 tablespoon olive oil

- Salt and pepper

- 1 large zucchini, sliced into coins

- 2 tablespoons fresh lemon juice

- ½ cup chopped mango

- ¼ cup fresh chopped cilantro

- 1 teaspoon lemon zest

- ½ cup canned coconut milk

Directions:

1. Preheat a grill pan, and sprinkle it with cooking spray liberally.

2. Brush with olive oil to the salmon and season with salt and pepper.

3. Apply lemon juice to the zucchini, and season with salt and pepper.

4. Put the zucchini and salmon fillets on the grill pan.

5. Cook for 5 minutes then turn all over and cook for another 5 minutes.

6. Combine the remaining ingredients in a blender and combine to create a sauce.

7. Serve the side-drizzled salmon filets with mango sauce and zucchini.

Nutrition:

- Calories: 350 kcal

- Fat: 21.5g

- Protein: 35g

- Carbohydrates: 8g

- Sugar: 2g

- Net Carbs: 6g

20. Slow-Cooker Pot Roast with Green Beans

Preparation Time: 10 minutes

Cooking Time: 8 hours

Servings: 8

Ingredients:

- 2 medium stalks celery, sliced
- 1 medium yellow onion, chopped
- 1 (3 pounds) boneless beef chuck roast
- Salt and pepper
- ¼ cup beef broth
- 2 tablespoons Worcestershire sauce
- 4 cups green beans, trimmed
- 2 tablespoons cold butter, chopped

Directions:

1. In a slow-cooking dish, add the celery and onion.
2. Put the frying pan on top and season with salt and pepper.
3. Whisk the beef broth and the Worcestershire sauce together then pour in.
4. Cover and cook for 8 hours on low heat, until the beef is very tender.

5. Bring the beef off on a cutting board and cut it into chunks.

6. Return the beef to the slow cooker and add the chopped butter and the beans.

7. Cover and cook for 20 to 30 minutes on warm, until the beans are tender.

Nutrition:

- Calories: 375 kcal

- Fat: 13.5g

- Protein: 53g

- Carbohydrates: 6g

- Fiber: 2 g

- Net Carbs: 4 g

21. Beef and Broccoli Stir-Fry

Preparation Time: 20 minutes

Cooking Time: 15 minutes

Servings: 4

Ingredients:

- ¼ cup soy sauce
- 1 tablespoon sesame oil
- 1 teaspoon garlic chili paste
- 1 pound beef sirloin
- 2 tablespoons almond flour
- 2 tablespoons coconut oil
- 2 cups chopped broccoli florets
- 1 tablespoon grated ginger
- 3 cloves garlic, minced

Directions:

1. In a small bowl, whisk the soy sauce, sesame oil, and chili paste together.

2. In a plastic freezer bag, slice the beef and mix it with the almond flour.

3. Pour in the sauce and toss to coat for 20 minutes, then let it rest.

4. Heat up the oil over medium to high heat in a large skillet.

5. In the pan, add the beef and sauce and cook until the beef is browned.

6. Move the beef to the skillet sides, and then add the broccoli, ginger, and garlic.

7. Sauté until tender-crisp broccoli, then throw it all together and serve hot.

Nutrition:

- Calories: 350 kcal

- Fat: 19g

- Protein: 37.5 g

Fiber: 2g

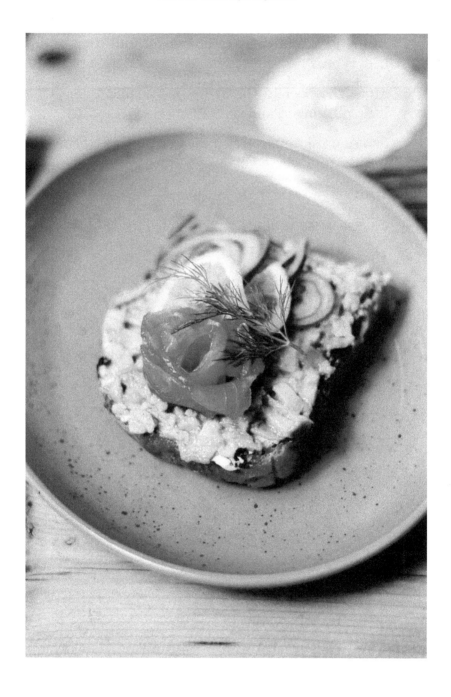

Vegetable Recipes
22. Roasted Mushrooms
Preparation Time: 10 minutes

Cooking time: 30 minutes

Servings: 2

Ingredients:

- 2 tablespoons olive oil
- 10 ounces mushrooms, quartered
- 2 garlic cloves, sliced
- 1 teaspoon thyme, chopped
- ¼ teaspoon pepper
- ¼ teaspoon sea salt

Directions:

1. Preheat your oven to 400°F. Spray a baking tray with cooking spray and set aside.

2. In a mixing bowl, combine the mushrooms, thyme, oil, salt, and pepper. Spread the mushrooms on a prepared baking sheet and bake in a preheated oven for 25 minutes.

3. Add garlic and mix well and cook for an additional 5 minutes. Serve and enjoy!

Nutrition: Calories: 157 kcalCarbohydrates: 6.1g Sugar: 2.5g Cholesterol: 0mg Fat: 14.5g Protein: 4.7g

23. Coconut Almond Egg Wraps

Preparation Time: 10 minutes

Cooking time: 6 minutes

Servings: 4

Ingredients:

- 5 eggs, organic
- 2 tablespoons almond meal
- 1 tablespoon coconut flour
- ¼ teaspoon sea salt

Directions:

1. In your blender add all the ingredients and blend until smooth. Heat a pan over medium-high heat that is non-stick. Pour two tablespoons of batter into a hot pan.

2. Cover and cook for 3 minutes. Flip over and cook for an additional 3 minutes. Serve hot and enjoy!

Nutrition:

- Calories: 111 kcal
- Fat: 7.5g
- Carbohydrates: 3.1g
- Sugar: 0.8g
- Cholesterol: 205mg
- Protein: 8.1g

24. Baked Egg Tomato

Preparation Time: 5 minutes

Cooking time: 30 minutes

Servings: 2

Ingredients:

- 2 eggs, organic
- 2 large fresh tomatoes
- 1 teaspoon parsley, fresh, chopped
- Pepper and salt to taste

Directions:

1. Preheat your oven to 350°F. Cut off the top of the tomato and spoon out the innards.

2. Break an egg into each tomato, bake in a preheated oven for 30 minutes.

3. Season with parsley, pepper, and salt. Serve hot and enjoy!

Nutrition:

- Calories: 96 kcal
- Fat: 4.7g
- Carbohydrates: 7.5g
- Sugar: 5.1g
- Cholesterol: 164mg
- Protein: 7.2g

25. Spinach Garlic Salad

Preparation Time: 10 minutes

Cooking time: 2 minutes

Servings: 2

Ingredients:

- 1 garlic clove, minced
- 8 ounces spinach, fresh, washed
- 1 green onion, chopped
- ¼ teaspoon sea salt
- 1 ½ teaspoons extra-virgin olive oil
- 1 ½ teaspoons soy sauce
- 2 teaspoons sesame seeds, toasted

Directions:

1. Boil four cups of water in a pan over high heat. Once the water is hot, blanch the spinach for 30 seconds.

2. Remove the spinach from heat and rinse in cold water. Squeeze out excess water from spinach.

3. In a bowl, add the green onion, garlic, oil, sesame seeds, soy sauce, and salt. Add the spinach and mix well. Serve fresh and enjoy!

Nutrition: Calories: 80 kcalCarbohydrates: 6.2 g Fat 5.4 g Sugar: 0.8 g Protein: 4.3 g Cholesterol: 0mg

26. Almond Peach Arugula Salad

Preparation Time: 15 minutes

Cooking time: 0 minutes

Servings: 4

Ingredients:

- 6 cups baby arugula, washed, dried
- 1 tablespoon water
- ¼ teaspoon pepper
- ½ cup almonds, toasted, sliced
- 3 ripe peaches, pitted and sliced
- 1 tablespoon balsamic vinegar
- 1 tablespoon olive oil
- Pinch of salt

Directions:

1. In a mixing bowl, add the arugula, almonds, and peaches. Toss well.

2. In a small bowl, combine water, vinegar, salt and pour mixture over arugula mixture.

3. Season with salt and pepper. Serve fresh and enjoy!

Nutrition: Calories: 152 kcalCarbohydrates: 14.3g Fat: 9.9g Sugar: 11.6g Cholesterol: 0mg Protein: 4.3g

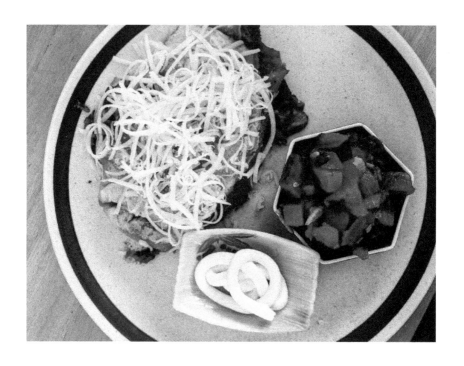

Poultry and Meat Recipes

27. Bacon, Beef, and Pecan Patties

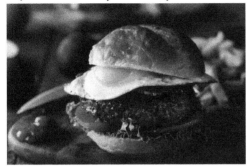

Preparation time: 10 minutes

Cooking time: 15 minutes

Servings: 8

Ingredients:

- ¼ cup chopped onion
- ¼ cup ground pecans
- 1 large egg
- 2 ounces (57 g) cheddar cheese, diced
- 8 ounces (227 g) bacon, chopped
- 1 pound (454 g) grass-fed ground beef
- Salt and freshly ground black pepper, to taste
- 1 tablespoon extra-virgin olive oil

Directions:

1. Preheat the oven to 450°F (235°C). Line a baking sheet with parchment paper.

2. Whisk together all the ingredients, except for the olive oil, in a bowl.

3. Grease your hands with olive oil, and shape the mixture into 8 patties with your hands.

4. Arrange the patties on the baking sheet and bake in the preheated oven for 20 minutes or until a meat thermometer inserted in the center of the patties reads at least 165°F (74°C). Flip the patties halfway through the cooking time.

5. Remove the cooked patties from the oven and serve warm.

Nutrition:

- Calories: 318 kcal
- Total Fat: 27.2g
- Total Carbs: 1.1g
- Fiber: 1.1g
- Net Carbs: 0g
- Protein: 18.1g

28. Lemony Anchovy Butter with Steaks

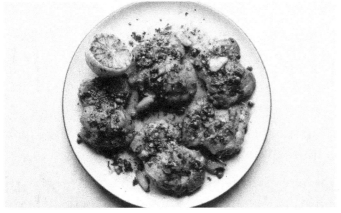

Preparation time: 15 minutes

Cooking time: 10 minutes

Servings: 4

Ingredients:

Anchovy butter:

- 4 anchovies packed in oil, drained and minced
- ½ teaspoon freshly squeezed lemon juice
- ¼ cup unsalted butter, at room temperature
- 1 teaspoon minced garlic
- 4 (4-ounce/113-g) rib-eye steaks
- Salt and freshly ground black pepper, to taste

Directions:

1. To make the anchovy butter: combine the anchovies, lemon juice, butter, and garlic in a bowl. Stir to mix

well, and then arrange the bowl into the refrigerator to chill until ready to use.

2. Preheat the grill to medium-high heat.

3. Rub the steaks with salt and black pepper on a clean work surface.

4. Arrange the seasoned steaks on the grill grates and grill for 10 minutes or until medium-rare. Flip the steaks halfway through the cooking time.

5. Allow the steaks to cool for 10 minutes. Transfer the steaks onto four plates, and spread the anchovy butter on top, then serve warm.

Nutrition:

- Calories: 447
- Total Fat: 38.1g
- Total Carbs: 0g
- Fiber: 0g
- Net Carbs: 0g
- Protein: 26.1g

29. Zucchini Carbonara

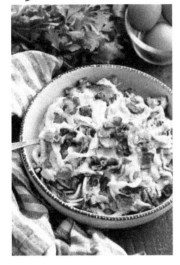

Preparation time: 10 minutes

Cooking time: 15 minutes

Servings: 6

Ingredients:

- 8 chopped bacon slices
- 2 large eggs
- 4 large egg yolks
- ½ cup grated parmesan cheese, divided
- ½ cup heavy whipping cream
- 2 tablespoons chopped fresh basil
- 2 tablespoons chopped fresh parsley
- Salt and freshly ground black pepper, to taste
- 1 tablespoon minced garlic

- ½ cup dry white wine
- 4 medium zucchini, spiralized

Directions:

1. In a nonstick skillet, cook the bacon for 6 minutes or until it curls and buckle. Flip the bacon halfway through the cooking time.

2. Meanwhile, whisk together the eggs, egg yolks, ¼ cup of parmesan cheese, cream, basil, parsley, salt, and black pepper in a large bowl. Set aside.

3. Add the garlic to the skillet and sauté for 3 minutes until fragrant, then pour the dry white wine over and cook for an additional 2 minutes for deglazing.

4. Turn down the heat to low, add and sauté the spiralized zucchini for 2 minutes.

5. Pour the egg mixture into the skillet and toss for 4 minutes or until the mixture is thickened and coat the spiralized zucchini.

6. Transfer to a platter and top with remaining cheese before serving.

Nutrition:

- Calories: 332 kcal
- Total Fat: 26.2g
- Total Carbs: 6.9g
- Fiber: 2.1g
- Net Carbs: 4.8g
- Protein: 19.1g

30. Mushroom, Spinach, And Onion Stuffed Meatloaf

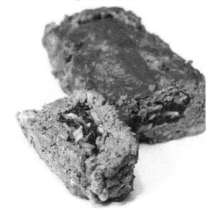

Preparation time: 20 minutes

Cooking time: 1 hour

Servings: 8

Ingredients:

- 3 tablespoons extra-virgin olive oil
- 17 ounces (482 g) ground beef
- 2 teaspoons ground cumin
- 2 garlic cloves, granulated
- Salt and freshly ground black pepper, to taste
- 6 slices Cheddar cheese
- ¼ cup mushrooms, diced
- ½ cup spinach
- ¼ cup onions, diced

- ¼ cup green onions, diced

Directions:

1. Preheat the oven to 350°F (180°C). Coat a meatloaf pan with olive oil.

2. Combine 1 pound (454 g) ground beef, cumin, garlic, salt, and black pepper in a large bowl. Pour the mixture into the meatloaf pan.

3. Make a well in the center of the beef mixture, and then scatter the cheese on the bottom of the well. Put the mushrooms, spinach, and onions in the well, then cover them with the remaining 1 ounce (28 g) ground beef.

4. Place the meatloaf pan into the preheated oven and bake for 1 hour until cooked through.

5. Remove the meatloaf from the oven and slice to serve.

Nutrition:

- Calories: 254 kcal

- Total Fat: 20.2g

- Carbs: 1.4g

- Protein: 15.3g

Appetizers and Snacks
31. Parmesan-Crusted Asparagus

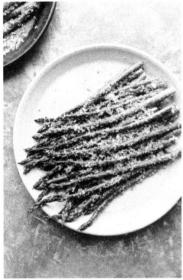

Preparation Time: 10 minutes

Cooking time: 15 minutes

Servings: 4

Ingredients:

- 1 ounce (28 g) shaved parmesan cheese
- 1 pound (454 g) thin asparagus spears
- 1 tablespoon extra-virgin olive oil
- Freshly ground black pepper, to taste

Directions:

1. Start by preheating the oven to 450°F (220°C).

2. Coat a baking pan with olive oil, then place the asparagus spears into the pan. Sprinkle it with parmesan cheese and ground black pepper.

3. Arrange the pan in the preheated oven and cook for 12 minutes until the asparagus spears are crisp and tender, and the cheese melts.

4. Remove them from the oven. Allow it to cool for a few minutes before serving.

Nutrition:

- Calories: 93 kcal
- Total Fat: 5.6g
- Carbs: 7g
- Protein: 5.3g
- Cholesterol: 6mg
- Sodium: 114mg

32. Low-Carb Cheesy Omelet

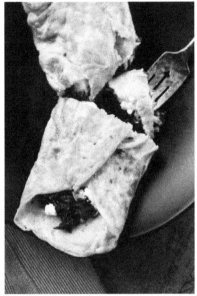

Preparation Time: 5 minutes

Cooking time: 10 minutes

Servings: 2

Ingredients:

- 6 eggs
- 7 ounces (198 g) shredded Cheddar cheese
- Salt and ground black pepper, to taste
- 3 ounces (85 g) butter

Directions:

1. In a bowl, whisk all the eggs until they are frothy and smooth. Add half of the cheddar cheese and blend well.

2. Add the pepper and salt to season.

3. In a frying pan, melt the butter over medium-high heat, then pour the egg mixture and cook for a few minutes until you see the eggs at the edges of the pan beginning to set.

4. Reduce the heat to low as you continue cooking the mixture for 3 minutes until it is almost cooked. Flip the omelet halfway through the cooking time. Scatter the remaining cheese on top and cook for another 1 to 2 minutes until the cheese melts.

5. Fold your omelet and serve while warm.

Nutrition:

- Calories: 899 kcal

- Total Fat: 79g

- Fiber: 0g

- Net Carbs: 5g

- Protein: 39.2g

33. Sweet Creamy Cauliflower

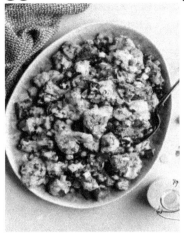

Preparation Time: 15 minutes

Cooking time: 30 minutes

Servings: 6

Ingredients:

- 1 large head cauliflower, cut into bite-sized pieces
- 1 cup shredded mozzarella cheese
- ½ cup keto-friendly mayonnaise
- ½ cup sour cream
- 3 tablespoons chopped fresh chives
- ¼ cup bacon bits
- 1 cup shredded sharp Cheddar cheese

Directions:

1. Start by preheating the oven to 425°F (220°C).

2. Put a steamer insert into your saucepan then fill the saucepan with water up to a level slightly above the bottom of the steamer. Boil the water.

3. Add the cauliflower to the steamer. Cover the lid and steam for 10 minutes or until tender. Drain and cool for 10 minutes

4. In a large bowl, mix the mozzarella cheese, mayonnaise, sour cream, chives, and half of the bacon bits. Add the cauliflower and stir to combine well.

5. Pour the mixture into a baking dish. Sprinkle with the cheddar cheese and the remaining bits of bacon.

6. Place it in the oven and bake for about 20 minutes or until golden brown and all the cheese melts.

7. Transfer to six serving plates. Allow cooling for a few minutes before serving.

Nutrition:

- Calories: 366 kcal
- Total Fat: 30.1g
- Carbs: 9.5g
- Protein: 15.7g
- Cholesterol: 53mg
- Sodium: 564mg

34. Faux Potato (Cauliflower) Salad

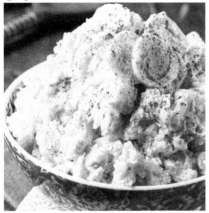

Preparation Time: 25 minutes

Cooking time: 10 minutes

Servings: 8

Ingredients:

- 16 cups (2080 g) water

- 2 tablespoons salt

- 1 (30 ounces/850 g) head cauliflower, cut into bite-sized pieces

- 1 cup mayonnaise, keto-friendly

- ½ cup thinly sliced celery

- 3 slices cooked bacon, crumbled

- 4 tablespoons minced onion

- 3 tablespoons unsweetened pickles, minced

- 1 teaspoon spicy mustard, or to taste

- ⅛ teaspoon ground turmeric

- 2 hard-boiled eggs, diced

- Salt and ground black pepper, to taste

Directions:

1. Prepare a pot of salted water. Bring it to a boil and add the cauliflower. Cook for 3 minutes or until the cauliflower is fork-tender. Drain the vegetable through a colander and set aside to cool.

2. Spread the cauliflower on a large platter and refrigerate for about 20 minutes.

3. Meanwhile, mix the remaining ingredients except for the eggs, salt, and black pepper in a large bowl. After 20 minutes, stir in the cauliflower and eggs. Season with salt and black pepper, and then serve.

Nutrition:

- Calories: 348 kcal

- Total Fat: 29.7g

- Carbs: 10.6g

- Protein: 10.6g

- Cholesterol: 63mg

- Sodium: 2001mg

Snacks and Smoothies Recipes
35. Stuffed Jalapeño
Preparation time: 15 minutes

Cooking Time: 0 minutes

Servings: 10

Ingredients:

- 8 ounces cream cheese, softened
- 2 tablespoons fresh chives, minced
- 1 tablespoon pimiento peppers, minced
- ¼ cup mayonnaise
- 26 ounces jalapeño peppers (pickled in a can)

Directions:

1. In a bowl, add the cream cheese and beat until smooth.
2. Add the mayonnaise, chives, and pimientos, and stir until smooth.
3. Fill each jalapeño pepper with cream cheese mixture.
4. Serve immediately.

Nutrition:

- Calories: 123 kcal Net Carbs: 0g
- Total Fat: 10.6g Saturated Fat: 5.3g
- Cholesterol: 26mg Sodium: 1,376mg
- Total Carbs: 5.8g Fiber: 2.2g
- Sugar: 2g Protein: 2.5g

36. Cheddar Biscuits

Preparation time: 15 minutes

Cooking Time: 11 minutes

Servings: 9

Ingredients:

- 1½ cups superfine almond flour
- 1 tablespoon organic baking powder
- ½ teaspoon garlic powder
- ½ teaspoon onion powder
- ¼ teaspoon salt
- ½ cup sour cream
- 4 tablespoons unsalted butter, melted
- 2 large organic eggs
- ½ cup cheddar cheese, shredded

Directions:

1. Preheat your oven to 450°F. Lightly grease 9 cups of a muffin pan.

2. In a large bowl, mix together the almond flour, baking powder, and seasoning.

3. In a small bowl, add the sour cream, butter, and eggs, and beat until smooth.

4. Add the egg mixture into the large bowl of the flour mixture and mix until well combined.

5. Gently, fold in the cheese.

6. Divide the mixture into the prepared muffin cups.

7. Bake for approximately 10–11 minutes or until the tops become golden.

8. Serve warm.

Nutrition:

*   Calories: 236 kcal

*   Net Carbs: 0g

*   Total Fat: 21g

*   Saturated Fat: 7.2g

*   Cholesterol: 67mg

*   Sodium: 165mg

*   Total Carbs: 5.1g

*   Fiber: 2.1g

*   Sugar: 0.9g

*   Protein: 3.5g

37. Crab Bites

Preparation time: 15 minutes

Cooking Time: 8 minutes Servings: 8

Ingredients:

- 1 pound canned crabmeat; drained, flaked, and cartilage removed
- 2-2½ cups pork rinds, crushed
- ¾ cup mayonnaise
- 1 large organic egg, beaten
- ⅓ cup celery, chopped
- ⅓ cup green bell pepper, seeded and chopped
- ⅓ cup onion, chopped
- 1 tablespoon fresh parsley, minced
- 2 teaspoons fresh lemon juice
- 1 teaspoon Worcestershire sauce
- ⅛ teaspoon hot pepper sauce
- 1 teaspoon prepared mustard
- 1 tablespoon seafood seasoning
- Ground black pepper, to taste
- 2–4 tablespoons olive oil

Directions:

1. In a large bowl, add all the ingredients (except for oil) and mix until well combined.

2. Make 8 equal-sized patties from the mixture.

3. In a cast-iron skillet, heat the oil over medium heat and cook the patties for about 4 minutes per side.

4. Serve warm.

Nutrition:

- Calories: 277 kcal

- Net Carbs: 0g

- Total Fat: 23.1g

- Saturated Fat: 4.1g

- Cholesterol: 73mg

- Sodium: 686mg

- Total Carbs: 2.2g

- Fiber: 0.3g

- Sugar: 0.6g

- Protein: 13.3g

38. Stuffed Mushrooms

Preparation time: 15 minutes

Cooking Time: 45 minutes

Servings: 4

Ingredients:

- 6 ounces clams
- 1 tablespoon butter, softened
- 1 tablespoon scallion, chopped finely
- ½ teaspoon garlic, minced
- 1 teaspoon dried oregano
- ⅛ teaspoon garlic salt
- ½ cup Italian pork rind
- 1 egg, beaten
- ¼ cup plus 2 tablespoons mozzarella cheese, grated and divided
- 2 tablespoons Parmesan cheese, grated
- 1 tablespoon Romano cheese, grated
- ¼ cup butter, melted
- 8 mushrooms, stems removed
- 2 tablespoons fresh parsley, chopped

Directions:

1. Preheat your oven to 350°F.
2. Grease a baking dish.

3. Drain the clams, reserving the liquid in a bowl.

4. In a bowl, add the clams, softened butter, scallion, garlic, oregano, and garlic salt, and mix well.

5. Add the reserved clam juice, pork rind, and egg, and mix until well combined.

6. Add 2 tablespoons of mozzarella, parmesan, and romano cheese, and mix well.

7. Arrange the mushrooms onto a platter and stuff the cavity of each with clam mixture.

8. Arrange the mushrooms into the prepared baking dish and drizzle with melted butter.

9. Bake for approximately 35–40 minutes.

10. Remove from the oven and sprinkle the mushrooms with the remaining mozzarella cheese.

11. Bake for approximately 5 minutes or until the cheese is just slightly melted.

12. Garnish with parsley and serve.

Nutrition:

- Calories: 331 kcal Net Carbs: 7g
- Total Fat: 25.6g Saturated Fat: 15.1g
- Cholesterol: 111mg Sodium: 644mg
- Total Carbs: 8g
- Fiber: 1g
- Sugar: 2.2g
- Protein: 19.2g

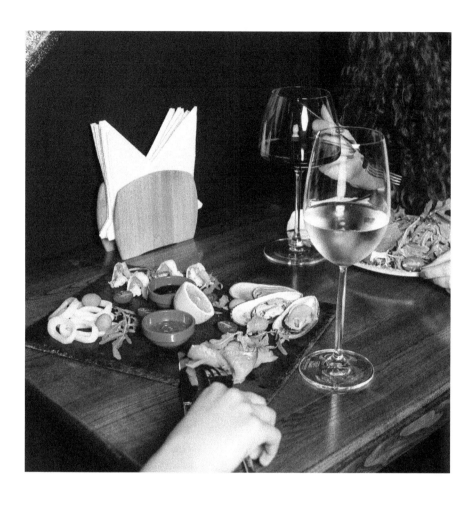

Desserts
39. Berries in Yogurt Cream
Preparation Time: 1 hour and 5 minutes

Cooking time: 0 minutes

Servings: 2

Ingredients:

- 1-ounce blackberries
- 1-ounce raspberry
- 2 tablespoons erythritol sweetener
- 4 ounces yogurt
- 4 ounces whipping cream

Directions:

1. Take a medium bowl, place the yogurt in it, and then whisk until it's creamy.

2. Sprinkle the sweetener over the yogurt mixture, don't stir, cover the bowl with a lid, and then refrigerate for 1 hour.

3. When ready to serve, stir the yogurt mixture, divide it evenly between two bowls, top with berries, and then serve and enjoy!

Nutrition:

- Calories: 245 kcalFats: 22g
- Protein: 4.2g Net Carbohydrates: 5g
- Fiber: 1.7g

40. Pumpkin Pie Mug Cake
Preparation Time: 5 minutesCooking Time: 2 minutes Servings: 2

Ingredients:

- 2 tablespoons coconut flour
- 1 teaspoon sour cream
- 2 tablespoons whipping cream
- 2 eggs
- ¼ cup pumpkin puree

Others:

- 2 tablespoons erythritol sweetener
- ⅓ teaspoon cinnamon
- ¼ teaspoon baking soda

Directions:

1. Take a small bowl, place the cream in it, and then beat in the sweetener until well combined. Cover the bowl, let it chill in the refrigerator for 30 minutes, then beat in the eggs and pumpkin puree and stir in remaining ingredients until incorporated and smooth. Divide the batter between two coffee mugs greased with oil and then microwave for 2 minutes until thoroughly cooked. Serve and enjoy!

Nutrition: Calories: 181 kcalFats: 12.1g Protein: 8.8g Net Carbohydrates: 4.6gFiber: 3.3g

41. Chocolate and Strawberry Crepe

Preparation Time: 5 minutes

Cooking Time: 5 minutes

Servings: 2

Ingredients:

- 1 ⅓ tablespoon coconut flour
- 1 teaspoon of cocoa powder
- ¼ teaspoon flaxseed
- 1 egg
- 2 ¾ tablespoons coconut milk, unsweetened
- 2 teaspoons avocado oil
- ⅛ teaspoon baking powder
- 2 ounces strawberry, sliced

Directions:

- Take a medium bowl, place the flour in it, and then stir in the cocoa powder, baking powder, and flaxseed in it until well mixed.
- Add the egg and milk and then whisk until smooth.
- Take a medium skillet pan, place it over medium heat, add 1 teaspoon of oil and when hot, pour in half of the batter, spread it evenly, and then cook for 1 minute per side until firm.
- Transfer crepe to a plate, add remaining oil, and cook another crepe by using the remaining batter.

- When done, fill crepes with strawberries, fold them and then serve and enjoy!

Nutrition:

- Calories: 120 kcal

- Fats: 8.5g

- Protein: 4.4g

- Carbohydrates: 2.8g

- Fiber: 2.7g

42. Banana Pancakes

Preparation time: 10 minutes

Cooking time: 15 minutes

Servings: 3

Ingredients:

- Butter
- 2 Bananas
- 4 Eggs
- 1 teaspoon Cinnamon
- 1 teaspoon Baking powder (Optional)

Directions:

1. Combine each of the fixings. Melt a portion of the butter in a skillet using the medium temperature setting.

2. Prepare the pancakes 1-2 minutes per side. Cook them with the lid on for the first part of the cooking cycle for a fluffier pancake.

3. Serve plain or with your favorite garnishes such as a dollop of coconut cream or fresh berries.

Nutrition:

- Calories: 157 kcal
- Carbohydrates: 6.8g
- Total Fat: 7g

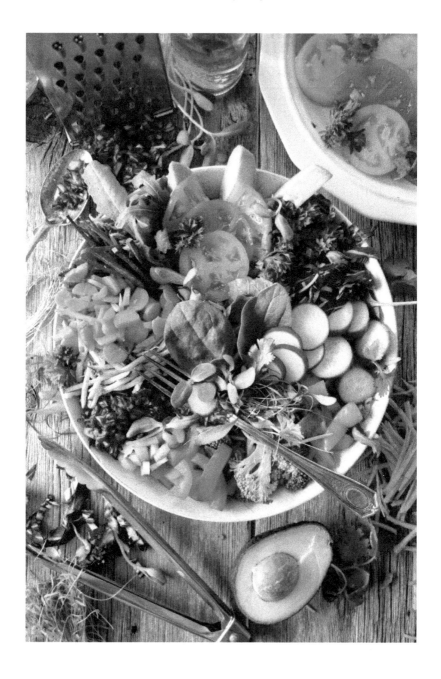

More Keto Recipes
43. Keto Ice Cream Sandwich Chaffle

Preparation Time: 5 minutes Cooking Time: 5 minutes Servings: 2

Ingredients:

- 2 tablespoons cocoa

- 2 tablespoons Monk fruit Confectioner's

- 1 egg

- ¼ teaspoon baking powder

- 1 tablespoon Heavy Whipped Cream

- Add selected keto ice cream

Directions:

1. Whip the egg in a small bowl.

2. Add the rest of the ingredients and mix well until smooth and creamy.

3. Pour half of the batter into a mini waffle maker and cook until fully cooked for 2 ½ to 3 minutes.

4. Allow the ice cream to cool completely before it's placed in the freezer. Freeze all the way to solid. Serve and beat the hot weather!

Nutrition: Calories: 158 kcal Calories from Fat: 141g Fat: 15.7g Sodium: 209mg Potassium: 128mg Carbohydrates: 9.9g Fiber: 2.9g Sugar: 0.9g Protein: 11.5g Vitamin A: 345 IU Calcium: 175mg Iron: 1.8mg

44. Pepperoni Pizza Chaffle
Preparation Time: 5 minutes

Cooking Time: 10 minutes

Servings: 2

Ingredients:

For chaffle:

- ½ cup mozzarella
- 1 grade A large egg
- 1 tablespoon almond flour
- 1 teaspoon oregano
- 1 teaspoon garlic powder
- 1 teaspoon baking powder
- 1 teaspoon red pepper flakes
- 6 pepperonis

For sauce:

- ½ tablespoon tomato paste
- 1 Olive oil light rain (to make the paste a little thinner)
- A pinch of oregano

Directions:

1. Mix the egg, almond flour, garlic powder, oregano, red pepper flakes, and baking powder together in a bowl.

2. Add the mozzarella cheese and coat with the mixture evenly.

3. Spray your waffle maker with oil (if necessary) and heat it up to its maximum setting.

4. Cook the waffle, check it every 5 minutes until it becomes golden and crunchy.

5. While it's cooking the chaffle, to make the sauce, mix the tomato paste, olive oil, and oregano. If your sauce is too thick, it will be helped by a teaspoon of water.

6. Cut the chaffle and apply the sauce to the tomato.

7. Sprinkle on top with mozzarella cheese and top with pepperonis.

8. Microwave to melt the cheese and cook the pepperonis for 30 seconds

9. Serve and enjoy.

Nutrition:

- Calories: 258 kcal Calories from Fat: 141g

- Fat: 15.7g Sodium: 209mg

- Potassium: 128mg

- Carbohydrates: 9.9g

- Fiber: 2.9g

- Sugar: 0.9g

- Protein: 11.5g

- Vitamin A: 345 IU

- Calcium: 175mg

- Iron: 1.8mg

45. Keto Cornbread Chaffle

Preparation Time: 5 minutes **Cooking Time:** 5 minutes **Servings:** 2

Ingredients:

- 1 egg

- ½ cup shredded cheddar cheese (or mozzarella cheese)

- 5 slice Jalapeno option-freshly picked or fresh

- 1 teaspoon of Frank's Red Hot Sauce

- ¼ teaspoon corn extract, is an essential secret ingredient

- Pinch of salt

Directions:

1. Preheat the mini waffle maker and place the eggs in a small bowl.

2. The remaining ingredients are added and combined until well absorbed.

3. Apply 1 tablespoon of shredded cheese to the waffle maker for 30 seconds before removing the mixture. It produces a very clean and friendly crust.To a preheated waffle maker, add half of the mixture.

4. Cook for a total of 3-4 minutes. The more you cook it for the crunchier it gets.Serve warm and enjoy.

Nutrition: Calories: 150 kcal Total Fat: 11.8g Cholesterol: 121mg Sodium: 1399.4mg Total Carbohydrate: 1.1g Dietary Fiber: 0g Sugars: 0.2g Protein: 9.6gVitamin A: 134.1µg Vitamin C: 0.1mg

46. Low-Carb Mini Pizza Chaffle

Preparation Time: 5 minutes

Cooking Time: 5 minutes Servings: 2

Ingredients:

- 1 egg
- ½ cup mozzarella cheese shredded
- ¼ teaspoon of garlic powder
- ½ teaspoon Italian seasoning
- Salt and pepper

Toppings:

- Tomato sauce, cheese, pepperoni, etc.

Directions:

1. Put all ingredients in a bowl. Mix well.

2. Preheat the waffle maker. When it's hot, spray olive oil and put half of the dough in a mini waffle maker or put all of the dough in a large waffle maker. Cook each chaffle for 2-4 minutes.

3. Add the toppings and bake or fry the mini pizza until the cheese topping has melted.

4. Serve and enjoy!

Nutrition: Calories: 118 kcalCalories from Fat: 72g Fat: 8g Sodium: 207mg Potassium: 52mg Carbohydrates: 1g Fiber: 0.5g Sugar: 1gProtein: 9g Vitamin A: 308IU Calcium: 162mg Iron: 1mg

47. Keto Chaffle Tacos

Preparation Time: 5 minutes

Cooking Time: 5 minutes

Servings: 2

Ingredients:

- ½ cup cheese cheddar or mozzarella cheese, shredded
- 1 egg
- ¼ teaspoon Italian seasoning
- 1 pound ground beef octopus seasoning ingredients
- 1 teaspoon chili powder
- 1 teaspoon cumin
- ½ teaspoon garlic powder
- ½ teaspoon cocoa powder
- ¼ teaspoon onion powder
- ¼ teaspoon salt
- 1/12 teaspoon smoked paprika

Taco meat seasoning for large lots

- ¼ cup chili powder
- ¼ cup grand cumin
- 2 tablespoons garlic powder
- 2 tablespoons cocoa powder
- 1 tablespoon onion powder

- 1 tablespoon

- 1 teaspoon smoked paprika

Directions:

1. Cook the minced meat first.

2. Add all taco meat seasonings. Cocoa powder is optional, but completely enhances the flavor of all the other seasonings.

3. While making the octopus meat, start making the keto chaffle.

4. Preheat the waffle maker. I am using a mini waffle maker.

5. First, whip the eggs in a small bowl.

6. Add shredded cheese and seasonings.

7. Put half of the chaffle mixture into a mini waffle maker and cook for about 3-4 minutes.

8. Cook the second half of the mixture repeatedly to make a second chaffle.

9. Add warm taco meat to the octopus chaffle.

10. Top it with lettuce, tomato, and cheese, and serve warm!

Nutrition: Calories: 118 kcalCalories from Fat: 141g Fat: 15.7g Sodium: 209mg Potassium: 128mg Carbohydrate: 9.9g Fiber: 2.9g Sugar: 0.9g Protein: 11.5g Vitamin A: 345 IU Calcium: 175mg Iron: 1.8mg

48. Bone Broth

Preparation Time: 10 minutes

Cooking Time: 10 minutes

Servings: 6

Ingredients:

- 500 g bovine bones (definitely also marrow bones)
- Liters of water
- 1 tablespoon of apple cider vinegar (optional)
- 1 pinch sea salt (optional)
- 1 bunch of soup vegetables
- 1 carrot
- 1 garlic clove
- 1 fresh onion
- 1 piece of ginger
- 1 teaspoon nutmeg (optional)

Directions:

1. Peel the carrot and onions and cut them into chunks. Wash the soup vegetables (celeriac, leeks, parsley) and cut into coarse pieces. Peel garlic and crush. Peel ginger and cut roughly.

2. Place the bones in a large saucepan and fry without fat.

3. Add the pre-cut vegetables to the bones and continue to roast together.

4. Fill the bones and vegetables with filtered water until everything is covered. Add 1 tablespoon of apple cider vinegar and parsley and bring to a boil.

5. Simmer for 3-4 hours. After 2-3 hours, if necessary, remove the marrow from the bones (continue to use) and continue to boil.

6. Bone broth through a sieve into another pot, season with coarse sea salt and other spices.

7. Divided it and freeze it or serve immediately:

Nutrition:

- Calories: 41 kcal
- Total Fat: 0.3g
- Cholesterol: 2.5mg
- Sodium: 486mg
- Potassium 24mg
- Total Carbohydrates: 0.6g
- Sugars: 0.5g
- Protein: 9.4g
- Vitamin A
- Vitamin C
- Calcium

49. Keto Chaffle Stuffing

Preparation Time: 20 minutes

Cooking Time: 40 minutes

Servings: 4

Ingredients:

Basic chaffle ingredients

- ½ cup cheese mozzarella, cheddar cheese, or a combination of both
- 2 eggs
- ¼ teaspoon of garlic powder
- ½ teaspoon onion powder
- ½ teaspoon dried chicken seasoning
- ¼ teaspoon salt
- ¼ teaspoon pepper

Ingredients for filling

- 1 diced onion
- 2 celery stems
- 4 ounces mushrooms diced
- 4 cups butter for sautéing
- 3 eggs

Directions:

1. First, make a chaffle. This recipe makes four mini-chaffle.

2. Preheat mini waffle iron.

3. Preheat the oven to 350°F.

4. In a medium bowl, mix the chaffle ingredients.

5. Pour ¼ of the mixture into a mini waffle maker and cook each chaffle for about 4 minutes each.

6. When they are all cooked, set aside.

7. In a small skillet, fry the onions, celery, and mushrooms until soft.

8. In a separate bowl, split the chaffle into small pieces and add sautéed vegetables and three eggs. Mix until the ingredients are completely blended.

9. Add the mixture of fillings to a small casserole dish (about 4x4) and bake at 350°F for about 30-40 minutes.

Nutrition:

- Calories: 229 kcal Total Fat: 17.6g
- Cholesterol: 265.6mg
- Sodium: 350mg
- Total Carbohydrate: 4.6g
- Dietary Fiber: 1.1g
- Sugars: 2g
- Protein: 13.7g
- Vitamin A: 217.2 µg
- Vitamin C: 2.4mg

50. Keto Chaffle Breakfast Sandwich
Preparation Time: 10 minutes

Cooking Time: 10 minutes

Servings: 6

Ingredients:

- Two large eggs, split

- ½ cup minced mozzarella or hard cheese

- ¼ cup almond flour (optional)

- 2 slice bacon (60 g/2.1 ounces)

- 1 slice of tomato (27 g/1 ounce)

- Sliced cheese such as cheddar cheese (28 g/1 ounce)

Directions:

1. Preheat the mini waffle iron. Whisk one of the eggs in a small bowl. If necessary, add almond flour and mix well. If only eggs are used, the dough will be very smooth.

2. Sprinkle a quarter of the minced mozzarella cheese (about ½ ounces/14 g) on a waffle iron and sprinkle half of the whipped egg on top. Alternatively, whisk eggs directly with mozzarella cheese.

3. Sprinkle a quarter more of mozzarella (about ½ ounces/14 g) and close the iron. Cook for 2-3 minutes until the waffles come off easily. Repeat for the second waffle.

Keto chaffle breakfast sandwich

1. Cook the bacon slices in a small skillet and scramble the remaining eggs in the same skillet.

2. Put on top of the waffles some sliced cheese, tomatoes, bacon, and eggs, finish with another waffle on top and serve.

Nutrition:

- Energy (calories): 58 kcal

- Protein: 4.55 g

- Fat: 4.19 g

- Carbohydrates: 0.61 g

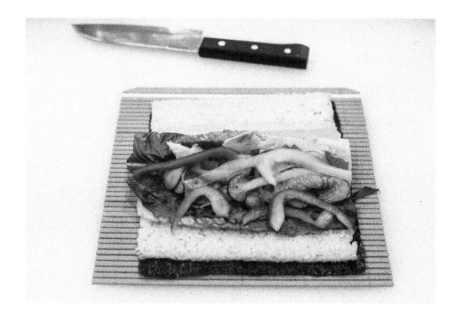

Conclusion

Thank you for making it through the end. Taking your first steps towards a healthy life is probably one of the hardest and bravest things a person can do. By choosing to follow a ketogenic diet, you are taking that challenging first step. Use the information you have learned throughout this book to help make this transition easier and more fulfilling. Just know that it doesn't matter how old you are, how big you are, or how physically active you are, because all of that can be changed through taking that first step. The best place to start off would be to figure out your numbers and then go through your house and start trashing the foods you will no longer have.

This is going to test you, and it won't be easy, but once you start seeing the results, it will be fulfilling. You will notice some quick changes, and while those may slow down over time, if you stick to the diet, you will see the weight fall off. It's easy to enjoy this diet, as well. The important thing is to get creative, and you will soon find that you can enjoy any meal you enjoyed before, but with a carb-friendly twist.

Ensure that you have your goals set and have all of the food that you will need to be successful before you start. Make sure you have lots of healthy fats because these are what will keep you full from now on. You can also play around with your macros to find that sweet spot that works well for you. The important thing is that you make this diet work for you. Now, go get started.

The first thing you have to do is write down the motivation or reasons why you want to change. This change must end at a goal. Wanting to lose weight isn't good enough. You need to be motivated due to the consequence of being overweight. Again losing weight isn't a clear goal. You need to set a certain weight you want to get to. You need to write it down legibly along with your reason. For example, "I will lose 50 pounds to help prevent me from getting diabetes." This is a great goal. Self-control and willpower can't happen until these other steps happen. Writing a goal along with two specifics and reading that goal every day will create a trigger by giving the goal specifics.

Lightning Source UK Ltd.
Milton Keynes UK
UKHW050441270421
382633UK00005B/24